# Your Amazing
## Itty Bitty®
# Self-Hypnosis
# Book

*15 Powerful Ways To Use*
*Self-Hypnosis To Improve Your Life*

Amy Mayne Robinson, C.Ht

Published by Itty Bitty® Publishing
A subsidiary of S & P Productions, Inc.

Itty Bitty® Publishing
311 Main Street, Suite D
El Segundo, CA 90245
(310) 640-8885


ISBN: 978-1-931191-73-9

*Dedication:*

*To my parents for all they have given me and my ancestors for their bravery; my husband, for believing in me and learning along with me; my daughter, giving me the chance to see intention come to life; My siblings and wonderful friends that always play along with my hunches; those many masters that taught me lessons; to you the curious, you will learn to trust own voice...you will find it! For my clients that trust me to guide them where they want to go; The Silverlake Reservoir Crew where this came to life; Dr. Mark, Tnah, Mario, Cheryl O', Dr. Kappas, Neale Donald Walsch, Emma Curtis Hopkins, Richard Bach, Emerson, H.M.I., Tim from A Better Living Permanent Housing and Support Services for allowing me to speak each week and motivate those whom have had a life shift; for Bill Lockwood you helped me find my voice. I'm grateful for the side of myself that is always yearning for more ways to find love in all I see; To Suzy Prudden for coming to life off of my bookshelf! For Joan getting this into physical form. Thank You All!!! Enjoy and always feel the Love!*

Stop by our website to learn more about Self-Hypnosis.

www.IttyBittyPublishing.com

or visit Amy at:

*www.Maynelypositive.com*
*or*
*www.Hypno4u.net*

**Skype Sessions available**

# Table of Contents

# Introduction

What is all this Hype about Hypnosis?
You might have an outdated version of what it is,
or what it isn't.

Have you ever put your key in the ignition or
lock without even looking? Have you wondered
why you missed your exit? Have you ever sung
along to a song you haven't heard in 30 years and
still know every word? Have you ever cheered
your favorite team on for a victory, getting so
wrapped up in the game you forgot everything
else? Have you fallen in love so completely you
lost track other important events?

These are all a type of Hypnosis. So if you say
you can't be hypnotized...guess what? You
already have been hypnotized several thousand
times in your life. Now you can learn how to
harness this powerful technique to tune into what
you are seeking in life!

This Itty Bitty book will show you many ways to
tap into the powerful subconscious and help you
begin to get the life you have been imagining!

It will introduce and familiarize you with many
tools, such as:

- You can learn to switch off your remote
  control self that isn't working for you and
  learn to awaken to a new way of being in

areas that you have wanted to shift for quite some time.

- It will help you utilize your powerful natural abilities to create the life you have been seeing from afar. This book will help you navigate the waters of your mind and life.

Are you ready?

Of course you are! This amazing Itty Bitty® Book will truly launch you into a new transformation!!!

# 1st Powerful Way
## What Is Self-Hypnosis?

Self-Hypnosis is a focused state of awareness that
creates behaviors that eventually become your
second nature. These behaviors make up who you
are and what you seek to be in this life.

1. Have you ever zoned out?
2. Have you ever sung along to a song you
   haven't heard in years and still know
   every word?
3. Have you cheered your favorite team on
   and were so wrapped up in the game you
   forgot everything else?
4. Have you ever fallen in love so
   completely as to become oblivious to all
   other important events?
5. Have you ever had a fear or phobia or
   habit and can't seem to shake it?

These are all forms of Hypnosis; when your
automatic pilot, your co-pilot and your
subconscious kicks in and runs your life.

This Itty Bitty® Book will help you recognize and
begin tapping into those states and become more
aware of your behavior choices.

1

## Improving Your Awareness Tips

- Becoming aware of when you go into the hypnotic state.
- Learning what it feels like to be in this state.
- Claiming new ways of being.
- Seeing how often you go on auto pilot.
- Pulling yourself back to the now.
- Learning how much you can do with this new sense of wonder and empowerment.
- Seeing if your fears are really yours or were they passed onto you without your consent.
- Are you supporting things that no longer support you?
- Reducing stress by understanding more about the ways you have been conditioned.
- Making decisions that empower you in ways you have always wanted.

# 2nd Powerful Way
## How Powerful Is Your Subconscious?

Research and science have determined that you use 8-12% of your conscious mind power and the other 88% -92% is your remote control system – your subconscious self.

1. This is an overwhelmingly large portion of control. All of this was formed into your way of being when you were just beginning your life and while your brain was growing. In fact, most of your subconscious was set up by the time you were 8 years old. This was the time your beliefs were downloaded and your neuroplasticity was ignited and formed.
2. Imagine yourself as an adult trying to re-learn everything again, as you learned when you were a kid.
3. "Eat all of your veggies, look both ways before crossing the street, don't talk to strangers, you don't do that, you don't like this, but you do like that." What are your beliefs?
4. All of this information was absorbed to form you and your way of being.
5. Do you ever wonder what portion of your brain is being used and when?

## Improving Your Subconscious

- Establish what behavior you are seeking to change and become aware when you behave that way without any effort?
- What belief(s) are yours and which ones aren't?
- Make a list of the ways you want to change those beliefs.
- Is your child-self still controlling your desires?
- Get all of your senses on board with your new desire.
- Spend a few moments each day writing out the way in which you would like this new belief to come to life.
- Journal out any old thoughts that have kept you cornered.
- Spend time people-watching and see if you can spot their "subconscious" moments and traits.
- Become more aware of the triggers that bring your subconscious traits to the surface.

# 3rd Powerful Way
## Who Is In Your Driver's Seat?

By now you may have started to notice where
your 88% takes over or who is driving your life
bus? It is fascinating to start to uncover the ways
in which you lose your senses and let the 'Big
Guy" or "Gal" – your subconscious – take over.
Sometimes, you have no choice when it wants to
be the driver; like when you want to really stop
over-eating, stop being afraid of that *"snake"* or
pick up good habits instead of self-defeating
ones.  Sometimes, the driver pulls right up to the
drive-thru window and gets what it wants,
whether it serves your destination or not.

1.  Start to see how many drivers you have
    on board?
2.  Where do they want to take you?
3.  How many are serving your highest good
    at the moment?
4.  Are you able to turn it around without a
    fight?
5.  Do you need permission to go in a certain
    direction?
6.  What is your destination?

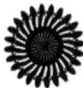

**Improving Your Ability To Take Back The
Wheel Of Your Life**

- When you find yourself making a choice
  toward an old habit, ask yourself who is
  driving? This will help identify and call
  out the pattern.
- Journal the powerful ways in which you
  want to steer toward your new goal.
- When you feel "power-less" lean into the
  feeling and ask what it wants you to
  understand.
- Before facing a situation that is your area
  of "weakness," put your most powerful
  self in charge. Then carefully plan the
  route that you will take to WIN just this
  one time! This will start redirecting your
  team.
- Once you have made a successful
  journey, the mind will start to understand
  you want more of that!
- Believe in your power and give yourself
  permission to claim all the GOOD.
- Destination is what you want to have in
  your life. Journal out those areas and
  make them come to life in your mind
  first!

# 4th Powerful Way
## What Are Your Hard-Wired Beliefs?

Understanding your nature/beliefs is one of the most powerful ways you can bring about change. When you are able to see beyond your current situation to your hopes and dreams, these are clues to what you are longing to accomplish.

Take a look at your Life Circuit Board. Can you see what needs to be replaced and possibly dusted off, or tuned up? Are you able to see if they are working for the life you really want to be living? Remember that 8-year-old you…is that child still running who you are?

1. Are your beliefs so rigid that your flexibility has rusted away?
2. Do they keep you from enjoying the life you imagine?
3. Are they from an outdated version of yourself, but they continue to influence you?
4. What could you use instead of this?
5. What would refresh you?
6. What would bring about transformation?

## Powerful Flexibility Within Is The Winner!

- Over a lifetime, if you won't allow for new ways of seeing, you will grow stale and predictable.
- When your dreams and visions keep knocking on the door to your heart and mind and you don't answer, they will eventually give up and go on to someone else who will listen and take action.
- Flexibility allows others to have their own mind, and you get to have yours as well!
- Finding out what makes you come alive is a true test of your beliefs...does it build you up or tear you down? If it is tearing you down, you may want to question if it has your best interest at heart.
- Try and replace the belief that is holding you back and rework it to a powerful "I Am" statement (i.e. "I Am Strong and believe I can make a difference.").
- When you tap into this part of your belief system that says, "I CAN Change," you are tapping into the transformational arena and the flexibility to win!

# 5th Powerful Way
## Your Intentions Are Your Map to Success

The word "Intention" is defined as: purpose, aim, and goal or end desire. If you can assess the power in which you listen to and live by intention, you will start to see where you are going and where you have been. Your intentions will take you to a destination; make sure you are charting the course to where you want to go.

1. Start with writing down your intentions. Take the most powerful one that is first on your mind, and then choose to see what it would look like if it were in your life right now.
2. Then write out a powerful sentence that spells out what your intention is.
3. Take the sentence to the end of it arriving and being in your life, RIGHT NOW!
4. Once you can feel your intention and it has power all around it, sit with this sentence as many times as you can throughout the day.
5. Intentions are the road map to where you want to go.

## Powerful Intentions = Success

- Intentions are a way of thinking forward from the end results. When you see the story ending in powerful ways and work backward, your defense mechanisms don't have to work so hard to protect you.
- Holding the powerful vision of what you see in your mind's eye from all of the good choices you made along your route lets your mind guide you with less effort.
- Sticking to a road map of focus helps get you there with fewer detours. Make sure your intentions are really the ones that you want now, right now in your life. You get to choose.
- Living from your powerful intentions, the mind has to figure out a way to get you there. Relax and let them sink way down into the core of who you are!
- The more connected to your core values, the more powerful the intention will be.

# 6th Powerful Way
## Change Your Territory, Change Your Life

When things keep repeating in your life and nothing seems to be shifting, it may be time to look at where, what and with whom you are surrounded. Are you being supported for your powerful intentions? It could be your environment and surroundings are keeping you stuck in an old pattern.

1.  Sabotage will happen if you keep doing the same things over and over, expecting (and getting) the same result. This is called madness. Breaking out of this takes noticing and allowing a new pattern to emerge.
2.  Check your territory. Is it supporting you and your powerful intention? You may have to shift that space to start seeing results.
3.  Examine your support systems.
4.  Are your intentions accepted and supported in the current territory?
5.  Do you want the change to happen? Resistance happens when you don't give yourself the right to accept what is yours.

**Powerful Ways to Claim Your Territory And Your Life!**

- When seeking to reach a goal you have placed in your sight, make sure you are heading in the right direction. This can make or break you. The right direction is empowering you to achieve what you are aiming for.
- Changing your territory if you don't feel strong enough to face the "Giant." This is where the path of least resistance comes in.
- Focus on your small successes at first. The day, the moment when you did something powerful to reach your goal. Then breathe that image in over and over.
- Keep your powerful intentions to only those that BELIEVE in you. Others will want to keep you in their territory for as long as they can disempower you.
- You will get stronger, just like an athlete, as you master and prove to yourself that you can have change happen in your life.
- Look for and focus on the good feelings of your new territory, even if you stay in the same exact spot. You will be different!
- Always keep your intentions list with you and see it coming true in many ways you may not have imagined!

# 7th Powerful Way
## Visualize and Imagine

It may seem childish to do, but somewhere along the line, you stopped using your imagination to hold great visions about life. Now is the time to take back that creative energy and foster its growth in you and in your life!

1. The mind uses images to determine what we like and what we dislike. Start focusing on the things you like!
2. Daydreaming got a bad rap! Try taking a few moments and let your mind drift to happy, empowering ideas of what your changed life and intentions would be like.
3. Make a list of words that have a visual meaning behind them. Keep this list near your work space and look at it a few times a day and your mind will start connecting the dots to your road map of success!
4. Images have great power and will accelerate a feeling within you to all of your cells. Choose your images wisely.
5. Play a game of imagination and strengthen your mind and the new connections you are beginning to form.

**Powerful Images and Creativity**

- Treasure mapping is a powerful way to get your mind into believing your new intention and your new way of being.
- Pick photos that empower you. Take a snap shot on your phone and have a slide show handy of your favorite images. By having your mind focus on this slideshow, it will impress your subconscious of your desires. Play this when your mind starts to drift to a lower vibrational state.
- Day dreaming is great! Take as little as 3-minutes and let your mind go to your favorites images. Just remind yourself this is creating new pathways to help you get your goal achieved. Direct them to only go to powerful images that float up. All others can be blown away on your exhale.
- The visual word list is vital to write out with your own handwriting! This is an ideomotor tool and uses portions of your brain to access powerful words and create feelings that you resonate to.
- Our cellular levels respond to images. Pick the photos that bring about a state of the most powerful feelings.
- Brain games will help loosen up the plaque buildup of complicity. There are numerous sites online that do this.

# 8<sup>th</sup> Powerful Way
## Create Your Future With Your Words

Words are the first powerful way by which you can shift up to a better vibration. Think of what you say as your script for life. Whatever you say out loud and repeat is what will happen in your outer life. Choose them with direct intention this will bring you the life you desire.

1. Check your script.
2. Are you on repeat and playing the same scene out over and over?
3. Use new words that describe the effect you are looking for.
4. What are you filling your mind with?
5. What are you allowing into your script?

## Powerful Ways To Edit Your Life Script

- Take a look at the "script" of your life and see if it is showing up with the power you want it to.
- If you are repeating patterns over and over, write them down and decide what pattern you would rather have instead? Then take the new pattern and practice saying your new script over and over in an affirmative and positive way.
- Grab an old fashioned dictionary or thesaurus and start looking up new words to use to describe the way you want to feel. This will retrain your brain to create new neuropathways!
- Do a check of what you are filling your tank with. Are you taking in too much negative? Negative thoughts, situations, media and even people will leave you running out of gas. Switch over to positive thoughts and watch your gauge soar upwards!
- If your life is throwing you situations that are draining you, double check to make sure you are only catching the ones that belong to you. If you try to catch all the "balls" that get thrown at you, you can get drained. Check your catcher's mitt. Make sure you are only catching those situations that help you win!

# 9th Powerful Way
## Upgrade Your Operating System (Subconscious)

Think of your subconscious as your operating system, your hard drive. Those long held beliefs that are no longer helping you get where you want to be in life.

1. Your operating system/subconscious will deliver what you fill up with the most.
2. Self-Hypnosis can be a great tool to bypass the stubborn ways that keep you spiraling out of control.
3. You have the power to change your thought once you recognize the thought that needs to be changed.
4. Research is suggesting Hypnosis is a great tool to calm your system and a calm system meets less resistance to change.
5. Spend a few moments a day noticing the ways in which you see old patterns that need to go.

## Powerful Ways to Upgrade your Subconscious

- What do you repeat over and over to yourself all day? Is it self-defeating? Begin telling that thought, you hear it and then switch to a better, more empowering thought (it will listen).
- In Self-Hypnosis, getting very relaxed allows the subtle changes to easily take place by not sending the flight fight reaction into action to take over.
- Come up with the powerful feeling of the new thought you would like to experience. Then start telling your subconscious to go find it. It will surprise you in ways you weren't expecting.
- Each and every time the old thought shows up, snap your fingers and replace it with the new empowering thought.
- Relax into the letting go and settling into the successful new habit. Give it room to come to life in your mind, and then it will come to life in your reality.

# 10th Powerful Way
## Change Mantra

Your mantra is what you seem to say over and over in certain situations throughout your life. Most are done unconsciously and can be very disempowering. Calling out this one element can bring a new awareness and more power to your focus.

1. Finding out what you automatically say can be tricky. You may have to ask someone what they hear you say repeatedly.
2. Once you identify your catch-phrase, count how many times a day you might say it.
3. Is it geared toward the negative?
4. Is it filler to keep you from tuning into something else?
5. Notice other people's catch phrases and you'll begin to see how such phrases can limit your growth.
6. Is it something you do when you get nervous? Or is it simply a habit?

## Powerful Mantras

- Create a saying that keeps you powered up.
- What would you like to hear the most from others? "You are doing a great job!" "Way to go!" "You are so brilliant!"
- Program your cell phone to call you by your new mantra. This is a great way of delivering Self-Hypnosis.
- Choose what you want to call yourself from now on when talking to yourself. It is healthy after all!…This can be fun and a great game changer. Pick something empowering!
- Think of yourself as the CEO of your life. Think about the way you would speak to your Board of Directors.
- Notice each time you slip back to your old mantra and see the difference.
- New mantras will be accepted and anchored in hypnosis as well.

# 11<sup>th</sup> Powerful Way
## Relaxation Techniques

Self-Hypnosis works best when you are powerfully calm and in a state of relaxation. It can be challenging to find those moments to unplug from our stresses and you may not know how to unwind. Here are a few of my favorite ways to settle into a great state easy and effortlessly.

1. Progressive all over body relaxation technique.
2. Breathing practices.
3. Sound journeys.
4. Reframing your thoughts.
5. Turning the volume down on reoccurring negative thoughts.
6. Imagery journeys are very powerful.

**Powerful Relaxation Tips**

- Progressive Relaxations start at the top or bottom of your body and unwind gently with a nice soothing color that brings you relaxation. Allow each body part to be filled up with this color – letting go and getting more relaxed.
- Breathing gets all backed up when you are in stress. Take deep belly breaths. Try and slow your breathing down to 10 or less breaths per minute. Try and see if you can get down to 4 per minute. This will detoxify your cells and rejuvenate your whole being. People forget the breath is the key to relaxation. It is always the first thing to check if you are getting stressed. Singing is also great for breath control and releasing tension!
- Sound Relaxation is becoming very popular. Binaural beats are terrific for healing and taking you to a deeper state of trance. YouTube has amazing choices for these. My website has a list of my favorites.
- Reframe Game. A technique I like to use to help create a lifestyle change is reframing a negative to something positive. This also helps lower your stress if you can shift it even in the smallest way. Have fun with it and see if you can start spinning it to the positive.

# 12th Powerful Way
## Entering the State Of Hypnosis

Welcome to the state that can transform your life!
You will get conditioned as you find the space
where you feel so calm and rejuvenated! It may
seem odd at first, but over time you will find it so
easy to drift to this state of awareness and
recharge your new battery that is leading you to
your newfound way of being.

1. Hypnosis is a natural state and you go
   back and forth out of this all of the time.
2. Sometimes you need to de-hypnotize.
   yourself before you can allow yourself to
   relax with this tool.
3. Work at bypassing your inner critic.
4. Turn down your defenses.
5. Understand your own suggestibility.
6. Decide what you want to tell yourself
   before you enter.
7. Learn to listen to the promptings that
   show up.
8. Learn where and when to use this.
9. As you awaken afterwards, you will
   bring new awareness back with you.

**Powerful Entrance to The Hypnotic State**

- Concentrate on one spot and gently bring your eyes to a softer focus, until the image begins to blur.
- De-hypnotize yourself to old patterns and beliefs; let them loosen their grip on you.
- Keep in mind what you are turning inward for…(Chapter 5 and your intentions).
- Follow your breath easily and gently and, if your focus gets pulled elsewhere, gently guide it back to the thought of your intention.
- Your inner critic may pop up from time to time and try to tell you lies about your goal – don't listen. Give your attention back to the intention that you want in your life.
- Your fight-or-flight defense may get triggered and try to get you to start doing something else, or tell you this will never work…don't listen, keep going and keep fully focused on your new intention.
- You are most suggestible to yourself! Make sure you are using the right script. (Chapter 8)

# 13th Powerful Way
## Allowing Change To Happen

You have determined what you want to change and now is the time to set all of it into motion. The power is up to you in letting a new thought take root and grow!

1. Keep seeing the new and powerful intention.
2. Believe it is on the way.
3. Understanding you're going up against old patterns.
4. Lean into the change.
5. Think of your new way of being as a seedling.
6. Make a quantum leap of belief!
7. Tell yourself, "I like it!"
8. Stay connected to like-minded supporters.

## Powerful Transformation Is Happening!

- Hold your sights to the new way of being, arriving and allowing it to grow in your consciousness. Then it will start showing up on the outside. The inside has to believe it wholeheartedly to be seen on the outside!
- Believe! Let nothing take you away from the certainty that it is arriving!
- If you always do what you have always done, you will always get what you have always gotten! Repeat over and over...
- Lean into the change. Do something that the new way of being would do.
- Think of your new powerful way as if it were a seed that needs to be nourished, like a master gardener would.
- "I like it"...tells your mind that something good is happening. Smile when you say it!
- Quantum leaps happen when you truly trust and see the power is within you and you can get where you want to go!
- Stay connected to social situations that believe in your new way!! You all need a good community...

# 14th Powerful Way
## When Will I Feel Results?

Change can happen in an instant. It is up to us to find out how long we think things will take. Once you know without a doubt, the proof will start showing up and you will feel amazing!

1. Stay in the NOW.
2. Create an anchor in your outside world, such as a small stone or trinket that you can hold onto.
3. Don't complain.
4. Hear the words, "You made it. Congratulations! You did it!!!"
5. Practice, practice and then let go.
6. Feel the end results with all of your senses. Get excited to the new way that is here!

## Powerful Results Equal Powerful You

- Stay in the moment. This will keep you out of the land of doubt! You are succeeding!
- Anchors are a physical touch that can remind you of your powerful intention. Small stones have a way of helping you focus on who you are and what you are becoming!
- Complaining truly puts all of your energy backwards. Catch yourself when you complain – this may be the hold up if you aren't seeing results. I love the "No Complaint Habit." Add this and you will see your results appear quicker.
- Be mindful of how long you held onto the old belief….give the new idea room to grow.
- Stay positive you are on the right path!

# 15th Powerful Way
## Is It Time To See A Hypnotherapist?

Self-Hypnosis is done with your own mind, your own power and your own words. A hypnotherapist can help you get to those places you might be holding resistance to. They provide you a safe and relaxing path to your subconscious and help you create the change you desire.

1. Resistance can block you, if the held belief is not willing to let go.
2. A hypnotherapist can determine where you might be meeting with obstacles you aren't seeing.
3. They are someone who has the tools to help motivate you.
4. They teach you how stay in control.
5. They provide tips on how to get to your results faster.
6. They foster new connections back to your powerful self.

## Powerful Ways A Hypnotherapist Can Help

- Resistance is your old friend; by talking it out with a trained professional you will clarify what has been holding you back.
- Most people think they will lose control if they are hypnotized; it's just the opposite, really. You learn how to gain masterful self-control.
- Trained hypnotherapists have lots of tools they can teach you to enter the hypnotic trance.
- The relaxation you get in Hypnosis is therapeutic and calming. This is where change can take place.
- Your owns goals are repeated back to you from a different point of view and sometimes, that is all it takes to get you back on track. Your power words are used.
- You will feel empowered and motivated!

**You've finished. Before you go...**

Tweet/share that you finished this book.

Please star rate this book.

Reviews are solid gold to writers. Please take a few minutes to give us some itty bitty feedback on this book.

## ABOUT THE AUTHOR

Amy has always had a gift of optimism, empathy and intuition, which led her to become a Certified Clinical Hypnotherapist and an award winning professional in her field. She is also a Certified Master of Therapeutic Imagery and a member of the American Hypnosis Association.

Amy lives in Los Angeles with her family and she maintains a private Hypnotherapy practice locally and also works with clients online. She loves metaphysics and has been a student of spirituality since she was in her teens. Some of her interest include The I-Ching, A Course in Miracles, Science of Mind, Neuroscience, healing sounds, angels, family, community, friends, good food, writing, reading positive books, poetry and lots of moonlight and living her life's purpose to bring love wherever she goes, is what keeps Amy full of life.

She is a sought after Motivational Speaker helping people learn how Self- Hypnosis can be used in their life. Please feel free to reach out to her to answer your questions about how Hypnosis can help you where you are right now.

Amy is starting a non-profit to help the homeless population. If you would like more information and ways in which you can help turn someone's life around, please check out her website.

www.humanity4homeless.org

Together we can help change the mindset and break the cycle of this epidemic.

If you enjoyed this Itty Bitty® book
You might also enjoy…

- **Your Amazing Itty Bitty® Heal Your Body Book** – Patricia Pinto Garza
- **Your Amazing Itty Bitty® Staying Young At Any Age Book** – Dianna Whitley
- **Your Amazing Itty Bitty® Cancer Book** – Jacqueline Kreple

Or many more Amazing Itty Bitty® books online today….

www.ingramcontent.com/pod-product-compliance
Lightning Source LLC
Chambersburg PA
CBHW060659280326
41933CB00012B/2241